10 Easy Ways to Change Your Life Style,

Your Weight, and Lower Your A1C...

Right Now!

Larry Oldham ended the threat of diabetes

with simple and straightforward lifestyle changes.

These simple adjustments to your life can save your life.

Defeating diabetes and pre-diabetes is vital to a

long and healthy life.

This book will help you accomplish the most important goal:

Keeping you alive.

*Other Books **by Larry Oldham**:*

EXPOSED - *Life Poems*

BROKEN HOMES BROKEN HEARTS- *Poetry*

THE TRIALS AND TRIBULATIONS OF BEING A WOMAN

A One Act Play

MAKING A LIFESTYLE CHANGE - *Health*

FOREWORD

A few years back my doctor presented me with the news that I was pre-diabetic.

He told me I have been warning you for years that your A1C was creeping up and you just wouldn't listen. Today you are at a reading of seven. That means that you are diabetic.

He gave me three months to bring it down or he was going to put me on pills. I did not want diabetes and I didn't want to go on pills. My only solution was to listen to what he told me and to follow his advice.

I started a regimen of daily habits that brought my weight down and brought my A1C down back to the normal level.

Will this work for you?

Maybe. All of it depends on many things: Your attitude, your aptitude, your perseverance, your willpower, and your openness to understand directions and to take directions to make you a Lifestyle winner.

He told me that 97% of the people who tried to diet and to bring down their A1C failed.

This book is not about diabetes, although if it helps lower your A1C, that is a great benefit to you and your health.

This book is not about dieting per se', although if you follow this regimen, you are going to lose weight.

Some of these habits I have been doing for years. I weigh every day. I have been weighing every day all my life. I will get into the reasons later, but this works for me. My wife has told me every day since we have been married that all the diet books say don't weigh daily, weigh weekly. Today she weighs daily and sometimes twice a day.

Losing weight is a mindset.

As my doctor told me, and I am sure other people have told you, it is a **LIFESTYLE CHANGE**. You have got to change your lifestyle habits to conform to a life that you can get used to, may not like, but will help you in the long run to stay the course.

We all want to live forever. This book does not give you the key to unlock that door, but what it can do perhaps is to extend your life by putting you on a road to better habits in your daily life. If the byproduct of changing some things in your life makes you live longer, hurrah.

I am the world's worst pupil. I don't listen well, I don't like authority, and I hate change.

Those three things alone should cause me to fail.

Something has to change in your life to awaken you. Something has to come along and convince you that HOW you are living your life just isn't working and you have got to make a decision to MAKE a change in your life.

My wakeup call was the A1C scare and the fact that I did not want diabetes; this made a difference in my attitude and my recognition of the facts. You might call it fear. You can call it what you like, but today my A1C is normal, I lost 35 pounds two years ago and I have kept it off, plus I ate birthday cake the other day.

Your reason might be totally different than mine. Maybe you want to attract someone at work, or school or church. Maybe you want to please your spouse.

Maybe you are just fed up with being the size that you are and you want a new look.

You can use any reason you like to adjust your lifestyle, but the most important thing today is to make that decision and to live with it the rest of your life.

Remember, that this is not the only way. You can take classes in Yoga for weight loss; work out at the Y or a exercise studio. You can read a million books on how to lose weight. You can go on a million types of diets. You can partner with a friend and help each other daily. All of these things will help you lose weight. Will they help you keep it off forever?

They might. If you find that that works for you, that is okay. I just happen to believe that after two years of making a plan and working my plan, my plan continues to pay off.

I am not smarter than you or anyone else. I am not a dietitian or a health guru.

I don't even believe in diets as a rule, because all of them I have tried have failed.

I do, however, believe in this **LIFESTYLE CHANGE** and if you will take the time to read this and then take the time to live it for a few months, you will find a new you with a new attitude and a new lifestyle. In other words a whole brand new you dedicated to the fact that facing your own reality and perception about your life and your lifestyle change, just may help you to live longer and look better. What a great concept.

WEIGH EVERYDAY

This is a policy factor for me. <u>WEIGH EVERYDAY</u>. Why should you weigh every day? Why shouldn't you?

Weighing every day gives you a road map of where you are going and where you have been. Your daily guide of how much you weigh is an indicator to your brain that you are eating too much, you are not eating enough, or you are eating just right. Knowing how much you weigh keeps you in line. If you weigh once a week and you have eaten too much you don't find out until it is too late. If you weigh today and you have gained a pound or two, this encourages you to cut back or at least be aware of the fact that you are eating too much. I would rather know what I did wrong today from yesterday than to wait a week to find out. It is too late at that time to do anything about it. I adjust my weight every day by what I consume. I have been following this pattern consistently for two years.

How it goes for me is something like this. I eat breakfast every day. At lunch I will eat something light most of the time, but sometimes I will eat a burger or a hot dog. This will make my weight jump up overnight. For dinner I might eat a meat and two vegetables or just a sandwich. The point is no matter what I eat today, by tomorrow I will know how my weight is affected by me weighing. I write down my weight every day also. This keeps me abreast of not only my daily weight but also my weight gain or loss per week, month, and year. Will this work for you? I don't know. I do know that the time it takes to weigh and the information that I derive from that knowledge keeps my weight in line.

Can weighing everyday have the opposite effect? The answer is yes. I do know some people that get discouraged when they see they have put on a few extra pounds and give up and start eating what they want daily. They are so discouraged that they figure this is not working so I might as well enjoy life by having an extra candy bar today or a soft drink or fries. It takes real will power to stay the course once you start this procedure. It is mind over matter as far as I am concerned. Try weighing daily. Write down your weight on a sheet of paper, a journal or an app. Plan your next day to compensate or adjust for the day before. One thing to be on the alert about is the fact that if you lost a pound the day before, or maybe with exercise you lost two pounds, don't overcompensate the next day and eat extra helpings of one more sweet as a reward. I do believe in the reward system, but I have a tendency to reward myself on the weekend instead of during the week.

I still weigh daily and I do a pretty good job during the week of keeping my weight in line. On the weekend I have a habit of eating things I would not eat during the week. This causes me to gain a few extra pounds on the weekend but because I weigh daily and I am aware I can re-adjust on Monday through Thursday of the next week by cutting down on portions, eating less fattening foods, and adjusting what I eat.

Weighing daily has helped me to keep my weight under control. It can work for you as long as you are aware of what your daily weight is saying to you. Be aware of the rise and fall of your daily weight. Adjust as necessary to keep or maintain the weight that you want to wear. Also remember that there are a lot more things in your bag to help you keep your perfect weight. We are going to address them in some of the next paragraphs. As I said before in my opening statement, being healthy, keeping your weight in line and living a good life takes practice, at first to adjust to the change in your daily routine, and then a change in your monthly and yearly routine, giving the **LIFESTYLE CHANGE** that I am talking about.

Can you do it? Sure you can. As I told you I don't listen, I don't like change, and I don't take directions well. I overcame all of my bad habits, made new ones, and now I am lifestyle healthy with new habits. All it takes is willpower and the attitude that you want to be healthy and look good. Isn't that what we all want in life?

WEIGHT LOSS APP

Ninety Nine percent of you have computers and most of you have smart phones now. One of the techniques of losing weight that I have found to be most helpful is the Weight Loss App. Most of them are free and some of them have better features, however you have to pay extra for the premium benefits. For me the free app works fine and I have been using the **Lose it** app for about five years.

There are many out there: **My Fitness Pal, Google Fit, Calorie Counter, Monitor Your Weight, Weight Loss Aid, Lose It, Weight Watchers Mobile**, and the list goes on and on.

The weight loss app is a tool for people who have trouble losing weight. It is basically an app for tracking calories to improve your eating habits. Using a weight loss app seems to make weight loss almost effortless. You will lose extra pounds using the app unless you cheat. If you are going to cheat about what you eat, exercise and how much you eat, you are never going to lose weight and if you do you will just put the weight back on in the future.

I have given you many brands to choose from and the one I like most is the **LOSE IT** app. As I said previously I have been using it for five years without any trouble. The app is motivating for me and I safely and responsibly use **Lose it** app to meet my goals. I wanted to lose 35 lbs. so I set that figure as my goal, put in the date I wanted to reach it by and the app gave me my daily calorie count so that I could reach my goal by the intended date. I did reach my goal using the **Lose it** app. You could set up a three month plan to lose fifteen pounds and if you follow the daily intake of calories you will reach your goal.

The **Lose It** app does many things. It gives you a daily and weekly average nutritional breakdown including sugars, fiber, cholesterol, as well as protein, carbs, and fat.

It gives you a record of your weight loss or gain and tracks your calorie intake. It is basically a food diary of what you eat daily. It offers you a database of food that you can search and even offers you grocery store items and all your favorite restaurant menus. It even has a bar scanner to scan your food item if it has a bar code and inputs the info into your **Lose It** app for the next time you want to look up that food item.

The **Lose It** app shows the total number of calories I've taken in in one day, the nutrition I have consumed from my menu and even how many days until getting to my ideal weight.

If you have ever had trouble losing weight, make sure to use a Lose weight app to help you reach your daily goals, and help you stay on course.

THREE MEALS / TWO SNACKS A DAY

Every diet book and every doctor will tell you that the secret to maintaining your weight is to eat three healthy meals a day and two snacks a day. Many health books will break this down for you and tell you just what snacks to eat, and what to eat for each meal. I don't object to that and I always say to follow the course that works best for you. You have got to remember that we are all different and everything that might work for me may not work for you at all. Also all of our bodies are different in some ways, our genes are different, our temperament might be different and the way our bodies handle food digestion might be different. Having said all of that I can only share with you the fact that this system I am laying out for you has worked wonders for me and for the past six months has worked wonders for my wife. We are both maintaining the weight we want to be and enjoying the food we love to eat.

I am not going to tell you what to eat daily, use your common sense. I am going to share with you in another chapter about eating palm size portions, but we will get into that later. Just keep it in mind while eating each meal.

I usually eat a regular breakfast consisting of eggs, bacon, toast, jelly and orange juice. Sometimes I might have waffles or pancakes with sugar free syrup or French toast with the same type syrup.

For lunch I might have a sandwich, chips, and a diet soda. I try to drink as much water as I can and most of the times use a sugar free powder to give the water some taste.

For supper I might have a meat and two vegetables, consisting of a yellow and green vegetable of some type. I might have a diet soda or water depending on my mood.

Here is the kicker though. I eat two snacks a day in between meals. You will find that also in diet books and I am sure your doctor has probably told you also. This is very important for two reasons. The first reason is it gives you an extra meal before eating lunch: taking away the craving that you are having by the time you get to lunch. The second reason is it takes that empty feeling away and by lunch time you are not as hungry and so you have a tendency to eat less. You can eat an apple or another fruit, or carrots or celery or even a pack of Nabisco crackers, although they are about 200 calories and 15 grams of carbs. You can do the same thing after lunch at about two or three o'clock in the afternoon so you won't be so hungry at night.

You have to be consistent in this and watch what you snack on. Be sure not to eat a full meal in between your full meals. The point is you don't have to diet hard or even cut out what you like at any meal or even at snack time as long as you count carbs and count your calorie intake by using your weight loss app and you will see the pounds drop when you weigh daily.

Do you see how this is working so far? Everything that I am telling you works together to make you more fit, keep your weight in line without having to give up the foods that you have always enjoyed. If you can eat what you want without having to buy special diet food and acquiring a taste for it, this plan keeps you in line without giving up the food you like. This system will work if you work the plan and stay with it. I promise you the lost weight without going on a "diet" will make you feel better about yourself and the control you have over your life.

WALK 30 MINUTES

<u>This one is a must be moment.</u> You have got to walk a minimum of 30 minutes every day. Some books say walk five days and rest two days, and other books say walk six days and rest on the seventh day. My doctor always says walk 30 minutes a day and I do my best to obey. I whine about it because we have hills in our

neighborhood, which is good for your heart, but tires me out. You can go to a gym,(I have done that, it was too crowded for me) or go to your park or track at your high school. The main goal is to walk at 30 minutes a day if possible.

Make sure your doctor is okay with this regimen. If you have heart troubles, leg troubles, back troubles or any physical impairment that dictates that you don't walk, then don't walk. But if your doctor says it is okay to walk and you can, you will be amazed at the results.

When you walk you are using almost every muscle in your body. You are moving your veins; you are getting blood to flow freely and at a faster rate than sitting. You are using your stomach muscles, your leg muscles to move you and when these muscles are being used there is less chance for atrophy.

Walking every day at least thirty minutes (I am now up to 50 minutes a day because my wife insists that we walk further) allows me to eat more of the things I enjoy. I honestly believe that the walking daily is what really brought down my A1C factor. I lost weight and with my lifestyle change of eating better and eating six times a day, helped me to get to my ideal weight, keep it there, and enjoy the same foods I had always eaten. Maybe less of it but at least I didn't have to give it up totally.

The other benefit of walking that you don't even realize is the fact that you are more limber. You can squat more easily or reach up or bend your knees without pain or grunting.

I haven't even mentioned the pleasure of the outdoor nature of birds singing and dogs barking, a neighbor waving. Plus you get to share time with your love ones if they are walking with you. Sometimes if I walk alone I listen to music or books on tape or motivational tapes about walking. Now that is funny. Seriously there are many benefits to taking a thirty minute stroll and once you get into the habit you will never want to give it up. It does rain or snow occasionally and you have to take that into consideration but it is not daily unless you live in a water zone or rain forest and that is the time you have to find an indoor area to walk in.

Two other things before we leave this paragraph. One is to choose your area to walk in. A safe environment is preferred at all times, so know where you are walking and who is around you. For me a flat surface on payment works and my wife prefers hills because she gets a more strenuous workout. Get a nice pair of walking shoes and wear them every time you walk. Dress comfortably with loose clothing or whatever you prefer depending on the weather.

The second thing is consistency. Get in the habit of walking daily to help you change your life. All of these ideas and recommendations are to help you make a **LIFESTYLE CHANGE**. As stated before all of these things work together to create your new lifestyle and help you better your life, with lower weight and better health.

FIST SIZE PORTIONS

What exactly are fist size portions and what does that have to do with me?

Fist Size Portions help you control how much food you consume. It is easy to go to a buffet and fill up on food. It is even easier to go to mom's house and have a second chicken breast or another helping of her delicious potato salad. All of that is well and good if you want to stay large, unhealthy, and not be a part of this lifestyle change we have been talking about.

You can eat just about anything within reason if you will eat in fist size portions. This doesn't mean a fist full or ice cream or as many donuts as I can get in my hand. This means eating what you want but only a fist size portion. The Bible says do everything in moderation. That is a credo I try to live by every day. Do I always succeed? You know I don't because I am human. I do try to do everything in moderation though and now that includes my portions of foods that I eat daily.

This is not as hard as you think. I have read some books that say order your meal at a restaurant, eat half of it and then take the other half home. I don't do this as a rule, however, because I eat a snack in between meals, I don't always finish my plate and sometimes I do bring a portion of the meal home.

If I am eating at home I try to eat the fist size portion to help keep me on my daily intake of calories. All of these ideas and suggestions work for me and I follow the carbs and calorie recommendations on my app. I try not to eat unhealthy foods, but eat foods that will benefit my body. I might eat mashed potatoes at a meal, but I will try to eat half of them if they are larger than a fist full. Remember you can eat just about anything you want within reason if you only eat a fist size full at one sitting. Without knowing it, these portions will more than likely fit within your calorie and carb count. The fist size portions and the fact that you have had a snack or will have one before your next meal keeps you from always having that feeling of being hungry and will help you maintain the healthy lifestyle you are striving for.

Get in the habit of gauging your food by size. Follow your app for carbs the calorie intake and stay within the perimeters of those guidelines and you will find yourself healthier and feeling better about your life.

SODAS, SWEETS, AND FATTENING FOODS

In a nutshell, don't eat them. That is really easy to say and easy to write. Living with all of the temptations surrounding us is very difficult.

We are subjected daily to the invitation of eating sweets. Someone offers us a piece of candy, or part of their dessert. Drinking just one soda a day won't kill you, but then you find yourself drinking two or more each day and there you are again over sweeting yourself. The brain is addicted to sugar. The taste of something sweet after a meal is a habit that we all have gotten into.

We all eat out at restaurants and how many times have you heard your server ask you *"Did you save any room for dessert"?* Their job is to sell you more food on your ticket. The higher your bill is, the higher your tip will be, is the way they figure it.

We all do that too. I find myself eating a lunch time piece of pie or some banana pudding or maybe just some ice cream. It is nice to get that greasy food taste out of mouth with something soothing like a sweet dessert. Those are calories and carbs that you do not need and just add weight to your middle.

If you are going to eat desserts, eat a half of slice of pie, or half a dish of ice cream. Eat a Snicker fun size bar instead of the regular size Snickers.

Everyone enjoys dessert or a soft drink. You can occasionally have one without ruining your diet. The main idea is to stay away from sweets as much as you can, and when you just have to have something sweet, make sure it is in a smaller portion or size.

Be aware of the fattening foods that you are consuming. Processed foods in restaurants have many calories and carbs. Use your app to see how many carbs and calories you are about to eat and make an effort to change the amount of food, what the food is you are eating, and ask yourself , do I need this, and how much do I need it, especially if it is not good for your body or your weight control effort.

All of us were raised on fattening food, sweets, and soda's. We are creatures of habit and eating is a happy time for everyone. Just be aware and try not to eat anything that is going to disturb your body.

You have instincts so use them. Use your willpower to beat the need to have a sweet roll or bread. Cut back at first as much as you can, and then if you can cut them back altogether would be your best policy. If this doesn't work just be careful to not overindulge on any one thing, or not overindulge on any one thing to the extent that you form a habit.

Choose a vegetable or a fruit for your snack or after dinner need. I know you have heard this a thousand times and I know most of you would rather have a sweet than a vegetable. Just remember you are trying to form a lifestyle change in your life and sometimes you have got to kick something out of your life or replace something in your life.

MAKE THE DECISION

This is going to be the hardest part for you in this presentation. We make decisions everyday of our life. Do I get out of bed, or stay in bed a little longer? From there is goes, what to wear, what to eat for breakfast, which way to work, do I want to work today, what project do I want to tackle first, what's for lunch, do I take my break now or later?

These are simple decisions that you make without much consideration. You just do them daily. This lifestyle plan that I am presenting you offers you the opportunity to turn your life around and maybe even extend your life by years. I can't make the decision for you and your friends can't make the decision, and neither can your family. If they love you they may want you to change, or cut back, or exercise more, or just about any reason you can think of to help you moderate your life.

Clearly, the decision to change your life rests squarely on your shoulders. It is your life. It is your body. It is your future.

Making a lifestyle change can be overpowering sometimes. We choose who to marry, where to live, do we have a baby or not and so on and so on. This decision about lifestyle is a major decision. If you are sick and not well, in debt because of doctor's bills, feeling lethargic all the time or irritable or mad because of how you look or your situation stinks, this affects all of those other decisions. You can't have a baby if you are not well. You can't buy a house if you have big doctor bills and bad credit. One of the biggest decisions you need to make is do I want to be healthy? What am I willing to give up being healthy, a few donuts?

This lifestyle change is serious stuff. This means changing your life time habits, be they good or bad. Your consumption of foods that you have always enjoyed, and has been your turn to meal when depressed, may have to change. This is not a quick one or two day effort. You are looking at changing your life forever.

I don't want this to sound ominous or threatening. I am telling you that with a little work and effort on your part, you can make this change. You can eat what you want, just smaller portions, you can still watch tv and play on the computer, you just have to work in thirty minutes of walking time.

So think about it. It was like when I gave up smoking. I gave up smoking three times in my life to prove to my friends that I could stop. Just as soon as I had proved it to them I started back. I went one year one time just to prove the fact that I could stop.

My problem was I never made the decision for me. I never stopped wanting to smoke so I always went back to smoking after quitting. It took my first son being born that made me throw that pack of cigarettes in the garbage and never pick them up again.

This decision is just as large. You have to make this lifestyle change for you. Your family and friends around you will benefit of course, because you yourself will be different and happier and they will like you. But in the long run you have to make the decision, give up some habits, do without some tasty treats you have always enjoyed and change your life for the better.

I only have one question for you. *ARE YOU WORTH IT AND WHAT IS IT WORTH FOR YOU TO CHANGE YOUR LIFE FOR THE BETTER?*

PARTNERING

Being married makes it easy for me to tell you to find a partner, or get a partner, or partner up with your spouse if they are willing. However, I do understand that some people live along, maybe in a new city and don't know anyone, or maybe you are just mean and don't have any friends. Okay, that was just a joke, so don't get mad at me.

All of this rambling is to tell you that if you have a partner, want a partner and can get a partner to change alongside of you, that this change is going to be easy. Maybe not easy, but certainly it is going to be easier.

I don't have to tell you the benefits of partnering with someone because if you have ever played team sports you know the importance of having someone who encourages you, or that you realize that person always has your back.

This **LIFESTYLE CHANGE** is the same. If you are both going through changes it is easier to talk to one another, support one another and encourage one another. You are both going through the same process and so you both can feel just what your partner is feeling. It is nice to talk it out and identify with one another. It is also better to have this partner doing all of these changes with you.

You can do it alone. In my case, my wife was already exercising, eating right and keeping herself in shape and her weight in line. She was always asking me to join her, eat more healthy, exercise with her, go for a walk with her etc. Sometimes I did, but most of the time it was easier to sit on the couch and read my book, or play on the computer, or watch tv even. Until I had my scare, and made up my mind to change my lifestyle, I was pretty much alone. As soon as I shared my problem with her she jumped right in and started helping me. Boy do I love my wife.

She started fixing meals that were low carbs; she started encouraging me to go a few more minutes on our walks. She encouraged me to walk up the large hills. Ugh! I hated those hills.

Quick story about the hills; *when I started my walking program I could hardly make it up the hills, especially the tallest hill in the neighborhood, which happened to be in front of our house. You couldn't go around it because it was the only way to our sidewalk. I beat the system though. Every morning I got into my car, drove down to the bottom of the hill, parked, and then after my walk, I would just get in my car and drive up the hill. How smart was that?*

She found out and she did not think too much about that idea. You need to walk the hills to get your heartbeat up, she said. My answer to her was that she would walk out of the house one day and see me lying in the middle of the road, worn out like an old mule.

Today I walk up that hill and don't think a thing about it. I still don't like it but I do realize the benefit through her encouragement.

There are many other benefits to partnering and it works both ways; she is now weighing every day. She is now joining me in an ice cream cone occasionally instead of being so hard headed about not eating anything sweet in her life because she might gain a pound or two. I have her using the weight loss app religiously and she tells me that all of these changes have made her lifestyle change much easier. She was already on the right track, but by changing just a few things in her life made dieting a little bit easier to take.

This is what partnering is all about; helping each other together to reach their individual goals through sharing ideas and suggestions to help each other be healthier.

It doesn't have to be your wife or husband. It can be family members, siblings, friends at work, neighbors. Just make sure you have the same ideas about improving both of your lives through changes that work for both of you. Keep focused on the goal, a lifestyle change to change your life.

STAY THE COURSE

What can make you stay the course? Staying the course means a commitment from you to work this plan. Is someone watching you and grading you to make sure you are on track? No, you are all alone on this journey and the only test is you doing the right thing to get the results that you want.

You can share this plan with your friends. You can give them the details of what you are doing to change your lifestyle. I don't tell everyone, but I do tell people that love me and want me to be healthy. For some, people partnering, or telling your best friend or a family member or your spouse may help to keep you on track to succeed. It is a mindset. It is a challenge to yourself that you want to do better. To stay the course means working longer hours at making this work, getting up earlier for that walk, making a conscious choice of what to eat and how much not to eat. What size portions and do you eat a dessert once in a while and if you do, how much and which one to eat?

All of the structures that I have presented will work. It has worked for me and for my wife for the past two years. We have learned to use these tools and procedures to improve our health. We have made the decision that we both want to live longer and share many more memories together.

Everyone has a different reason for everything that they do. Use whatever reason helps you to succeed, but make sure you stay on course to arrive at the state of health, that not only do you deserve, but a state of health to keep you happy and joyous in your relationships with everyone you know.

The other main reason to stay the course is just simply that you will be able to share this action with other people around you. You may save their life or at least extend their life by letting them know how you lost weight, got healthier, and had better self-esteem and more confidence in your daily life.

Staying the course means exactly what it says; choosing a better habit, changing that habit in order to make your life better. You have to decide that the effort you make is worth the value you receive by making that effort. This is not an overnight change. This is not an overnight success. This is a plan that has been proven that is effective and will give you better health. You have to stay the course to see the results. The best thing about all of this change as you will see is that this lifestyle will be with you for the rest of your life, your longer life.

Stay the Course and prove to yourself first, and to others later, that you have the aptitude, attitude, desire, willpower, and the knowledge within you to change your life through your lifestyle changes.

DO IT FOR YOUR HEALTH

In summation, I have laid out a plan that is very simple, has no downfalls, helps you be a better person, and gives you all the keys to changing your lifestyle to make you healthier. Give yourself three months following these examples as close as possible. If you do this without cheating yourself, several key things are going to happen in your life.

YOU are going to lose weight. YOU are going to change some habits in your daily life. YOU are going to be more aware of what you are eating, how much you are eating and why or why not what you should be eating. All of these suggestions are going to make you healthier. Name me one person that you know who does not want to be healthy.

This should be your goal, and to tell you the truth, this should be the goal of everyone you are acquainted with.

Make this change today. Make this a resolution in your life to better yourself through an action plan as I have lain out. After three months of enjoying changing your lifestyle, you should be excited for yourself and you should want to share this idea with everyone you meet.

After losing 35 pounds, getting my A1C down has only given me more confidence and the need to share this plan with my family, my friends, and everyone around me. Don't give up on yourself. Don't defeat yourself. Don't starve yourself. Learn to be healthier by changing your lifestyle. As my doctor now tells me; "I am not sure what you are doing but just keep on doing it because you seem to be in really good health."

Let me share this with you also. He tells me that I am one of the few patients that see him every six months and each time I have either dropped some pounds or have maintained by weight for six months.

All of the healthy tips and procedures that I have just shared with you, plus my commitment to change has made me much healthier. You too can be healthier by making up your mind to be in charge of your own **LIFESTYLE CHANGE**. Make that commitment today. Do it because you want to be happy and healthy. Remember this saying: **YOU CANNOT CHANGE THE WHOLE WORLD, BUT YOU CAN CHANGE YOUR WORLD.**

NOTES

About Larry:

Larry Oldham is an author, poet, playwright, motivational speaker, and artist who enjoys sharing his life with others.

He and his wife, Dena, write two columns a month, **He Said She Said** and **She Said He Said.**

The author of many poems and songs, he is the founder of **Evince Magazine** started in 1996 and still a flourishing magazine today.

His writing style is down to earth and easy to read.

You can contact him at **larry.oldham0@gmail.com**

Follow him on **Face Book/Larry Oldham**

Making a Lifestyle Change can be found on Amazon Kindle E Books.

What others are saying about this book:

I love your book, Larry. It's honest and really full of practical ideas. I'm admiring the progress you made with your life changes. I think you are right on target for the best way to achieve weight loss goals in a practical way. And, I think your ideas could be used by anyone wanting to make other types of changes in their lives.

A. Byrd

I think it's awesome that you want to help others who have received this despicable diagnosis! I pray that your book will guide many to a successful lifestyle change and good health!!

Darinda

This short easy read will inspire and motivate you to see the author's message re: the urgency of a lifestyle change. This book is a personal message about mindful eating and a healthy purpose driven lifestyle...why this is important and tips on staying the course. This book will make you Stop...Think...and Want to do it!!

Kathy Bullano, October 23, 2016   Amazon Kindle E Book Reader

I was given a copy to review. I found the book to be a good plan for fixing your "numbers". The steps when taken together will definitely make you feel better and have a better quality of life. It's a quick read and a good read and you can tell that the author poured his heart into the book.

By Aéyess, October 14, 2016

A very enlightening and informative perspective which can motivate the reader how to both manage and improve one's health as they journey through life. **Wayne Mobley**